MW01610277

Amazon.com/ author/ Jeanne K. Johnson

ISBN-13: 978-1517243760

ISBN-10: 1517243769

# Ketogenic Milky Strawberry

Total time: 5 mins

Serve: 1

**Ingredients:**

- ¼cup coconut milk or cream (60 ml / 2 fl oz)

- 1 tbsp MCT oil or extra virgin coconut oil (MCT oil is better as it doesn't solidify)

- ¾cup almond milk or water (180 ml / 6 fl oz)

- ½tsp sugar-free vanilla extract

- ½cup strawberries, fresh or frozen (72 g / 2.5 oz)

**Directions**

-Pour all the ingredients in a food processor and blend them till they form a smooth paste.

-Serve immediately by topping with some crushed ice and fresh strawberry slices.

**Nutrition per serving**

Protein: 2.5g

Fat: 27.4g

Carbohydrate: 4.6g

Fiber: 2g

# Smooth Chocolate Delight

Total time: 5 mins

Serves: 1

**Ingredients:**

- 2 large eggs, free-range or organic or 2 tbsp chia seeds or 2 tbsp coconut butter

- 1 tbsp MCT oil or extra virgin coconut oil

- ¼cup water + ½ cup ice

- ¼cup heavy whipping cream or coconut milk (60 ml / 2 fl oz)

- 1 tbsp cacao powder, unsweetened

- 3-5 drops Stevia extract

- ¼cup whey protein or egg white protein powder   (25 g / 0.9 oz) or 1 tbsp hydrolysed gelatine powder

**Directions**

-At first you will keep the eggs in the blender and then add cream or coconut milk along with water, stevia, ice and cacao and make sure to use the clear or chocolate flavoured stevia.

-Now it is time to add the MCT oil or coconut oil followed by whey or egg protein powder.

-Make a smooth paste and serve chilled.

**Nutrition per serving**

Protein: 34.5g

Fat: 46g

Carbohydrate: 4.4 g

Fiber: 2.7g

# Keto Vanilla Delight

Total time: 5 mins

Serves: 1

**Ingredients:**

- 2 large eggs, free-range or organic or 2 tbsp chia seeds or 2 tbsp coconut butter

- 1 tbsp MCT oil or extra virgin coconut oil

- ¼cup water + ½ cup ice

- ½cup soured cream or coconut milk (I like Aroy-D coconut milk) (115 g / 4.1 oz)

- 1 vanilla bean or 1 tsp vanilla extract (you can make your own)

- 3-5 drops Stevia extract

- ¼cup whey protein or egg white protein powder (high quality such as Jay Robb) (25 g / 0.9 oz) or 1 tbsp hydrolysed gelatine powder

**Directions**

-Start by mixing all the ingredients in the blender and beat them till a smooth paste is formed.

-You can use vanilla beans or sugar-free vanilla extract. In case you are using the vanilla beans, make sure to cut them along the length and scrape out the tiny seeds. If you want to avoid using raw eggs, you can use ground chia seeds to increase the thickness of the drink.

-Serve chilled.


**Nutrition per serving**

Protein: 34.6g

Fat: 45.2g

Carbohydrate: 5.1 g

Fiber: 0.5g

# Choco-Shake from Mexico

Total time: 5 mins

Serves: 1

**Ingredients:**

- ¼cup coconut cream (80ml)
- 2 tbsp (10 grams) unsweetened cocoa powder
- ¼tsp cayenne powder
- 1 cup water
- 2 tbsp extra virgin coconut oil
- 1 tbsp ground chia seeds (can be ground in a coffee grinder right before)
- ice as desired
- ¼tsp organic vanilla extract
- ¼tsp cinnamon powder

**Directions**

-Keep all the ingredients in the mixer and blend to make a smooth paste.

-Serve chilled.


**Nutrition per serving**

Protein: 6g

Fat: 52.1g

Carbohydrate: 6.2g

Fiber: 8.2g

# Smoothie with Blackcurrant (Ketogenic Version)

Total time: 5 mins

Serves: 1

**Ingredients:**

● ½cup blackcurrants, fresh or frozen (60 g / 2.1 oz)

● ½cup water (120 ml / 4 fl oz)

● 2 tbsp chia seeds, whole or powdered (16 g / 0.6 oz)

● ¼cup coconut milk or heavy whipping cream (60 ml / 2 fl oz)

● ½vanilla bean or ½ tsp sugar-free vanilla extract

● ¼cup strawberries, 2-3 strawberries, fresh or frozen (36 g / 1.3 oz)

● optional: 5-7 drops liquid Stevia extract or other healthy low-carb sweetener from this list

**Directions**

-Keep all the ingredients in the blender and make a smooth paste.

-Let the smoothie sit for a minute and then serve.


**Nutrition per serving**

Protein: 5.1g

Fat: 17.3g

Carbohydrate: 8.7g

Fiber: 9.4g

# Pink Colored Smoothie

Total time: 5 mins

Serves: 1

**Ingredients:**

- ½small dragon fruit (50g / 1.8 oz)
- 1 scoop whey protein powder (vanilla or plain) or egg white powder or hydrolysed powdered gelatin (25g / 0.9 oz)
- ½cup water
- 1 small wedge Galia melon (50g / 1.8 oz)
- ½cup coconut milk (or full-fat cream)
- 1 tbsp chia seeds
- 3-6 drops liquid Stevia extract or other healthy low-carb sweetener
- ice cubes (if needed)

**Directions**

-Start by measuring out all the ingredients and keep them in the blender.

-Make a smooth paste and serve chilled.

**Nutrition per serving**

Protein: 24.6g

Fat: 28.6g

Carbohydrate: 12.1g

Fiber: 5.5g

# Keto Smoothie-de-Pumpkin

Total time: 5 mins

Serves: 1

**Ingredients:**

- ¼cup pumpkin purée, BPA-free, canned or home-made (50g / 1.8 oz)

- ¼cup almond milk, unsweetened or pumpkin juice (60 ml / 2 fl oz)

- 1 scoop whey protein powder (vanilla or plain) or egg white powder or hydrolysed powdered gelatin (25g / 0.9 oz)

- ¼cup crème fraîche / sour cream / plain full fat yogurt or coconut milk (60g / 2.1 oz)

- ½tsp gingerbread spice mix (~ ¼ tsp cinnamon, pinch nutmeg, ginger and cloves)

- 1 tsp Erythritol (non GMO) or other healthy low-carb sweetener from this list

- 3-6 drops liquid Stevia extract (Clear / Vanilla / Cinnamon) or more to taste

- 2 tbsp whipped cream or coconut cream

**Directions**

-Keep all the ingredients in the blender and make a smooth paste.

-Serve chilled by topping with whipped cream and sprinkle with cinnamon.

**Nutrition per serving**

Protein: 21.7g

Fat: 17g

Carbohydrate: 6.6g

Fiber: 4.2g

# Smoothie of Leprechaun Protein

Total time: 5 mins

Serves: 1

**Ingredients:**

- ½average avocado (100g / 3.5 oz)

- 1 scoop vanilla whey protein powder (vanilla or plain) or egg white powder or hydrolysed powdered gelatin (25g / 0.9 oz)

- 2 tbsp pistachio nuts (unsalted) (20g / 0.7 oz)

- ½water

- ¼cup coconut milk, organic (or full-fat cream)

- ¼cup fresh baby spinach

- ¼cup fresh mint

- ice cubes (if needed)

- 1 vanilla bean (or ½ - 1 tsp vanilla extract

- 3-6 drops liquid Stevia extract   or other healthy low-carb sweetener

**Directions**

-Start by washing the mint and spinach and then cut the avocado into half and blend all the ingredients to make a smooth paste.

-Serve chilled.

**Nutrition per serving**

Protein: 27.2g

Fat: 37.1g

Carbohydrate: 9.4g

Fiber: 16.6g

# Smoothie with Kiwi Berries

Total time: 5 mins

Serves: 1

**Ingredients:**

- ¼average avocado (50g / 1.8 oz)

- ¼cup kiwi berries or kiwi fruit (30g / 1 oz)

- 1 scoop vanilla whey protein powder (vanilla or plain) or egg white powder or hydrolysed powdered gelatin (25g / 0.9 oz)

- ½cup water

- ¼cup coconut milk (or coconut cream or full-fat cream)

- 1 small wedge of Galia melon (or Honeydew, Cantaloupe) (50g / 1.8 oz)

- 1 tbsp chia seeds (or psyllium) - this adds thickness with no extra carbs

- 3-6 drops liquid Stevia extract (I recommend SweetLeaf or NuNaturals) or other healthy low-carb sweetener from this list

- ice (if needed)

**Directions**

-Cut the avocado into halves and then scoop out the flesh and then keep all the ingredients in the blender.

-Make a smooth paste and serve chilled.

## Nutrition per serving

Protein: 23.9g

Fat: 23.3g

Carbohydrate: 10.8g

Fiber: 9.7g

# Keto Smoothie-de-Horchata

Total time: 20 mins

Serves: 2

**Ingredients:**

- 2 handfuls almonds blanched (60g / 2.1 oz)

- 2 tbsp chia seeds, whole or ground (16g / 0.6 oz)

- 15-20 drops liquid Stevia extract (Clear / Cinnamon)

- 3 tbsp Erythritol (non-GMO) or other healthy low-carb sweetener from this list (30g / 1.1 oz)

- 2 cups warm water (480 ml / 16.2 fl oz)

- 1 cup almond milk (unsweetened) (240 ml / 8.1 fl oz)

- 1 tbsp lime zest (fresh)

- 1 tsp cinnamon (+ 1 piece of whole cinnamon stick)

- 1 large egg (free-range or organic)

**Directions**

-Keep the blanched almonds along with the cinnamon stick and fresh lime zest in a bowl and cover it with 2 cups of warm water and then let it stand for at least 8 hours. Overnight will be better.

-Now remove the cinnamon stick and lime zest and keep the almonds along with the water in a small sauce pan and add the almond milk as well as puree with a hand blender to make a smooth paste.

-You will have to heat this mixture till it starts to sizzle and then add the cinnamon and sweeteners.

-Now whisk the egg and pour it into this mixture and stir continuously to avoid any clumping. Stir and cook for a couple of minutes.

-Remove from the heat and mix the chia seeds and then allow the paste to thicken.

-Once the smoothie is thick, you will pour it into the glass and keep in fridge to chill and then serve.


**Nutrition per serving**

Protein: 11.9g

Fat: 22.2g

Carbohydrate: 5g

Fiber: 8.6g

# Rhubarb Pie & Strawberry Smoothie

Total time: 5    mins

Serves: 1

**Ingredients:**

- 2-4 medium strawberries (40g / 1.4 oz)

- 1 large egg (free-range or organic)

- 1 tsp freshly grated ginger root (or 1/2 tsp ginger root powder)

- ½tsp pure vanilla bean extract (~ 1 vanilla bean)

- 1-2 medium rhubarb stalks (50g / 1.8 oz)

- ½cup almond milk, unsweetened (120 ml / 4 fl oz)

- 2 tbsp full-fat cream or coconut milk

- ¼cup almonds or 1 tbsp almond butter (28g / 1 oz)

- 3-6 drops liquid liquid Stevia extract (Clear / Vanilla)

**Directions**

-Keep all the ingredients in the blender and make a smooth paste.

-Serve chilled.


**Nutrition per serving**

Protein: 14.2g

Fat:    31.8g

Carbohydrate: 8.6g

Fiber: 6.1g

# Ketogenic Smoothie with Peanut Butter

Total time: 5    mins

Serves: 1

**Ingredients:**

- 1 cup Coconut Milk (from the carton)

- 2 tbsp. SF Torani Salted Caramel

- 1/4 tsp. Xanthan Gum

- 7 Ice Cubes

- 1 tbsp. MCT Oil

- 2 tbsp. Peanut Butter

**Directions**

-Keep all the ingredients into the blender and blend them till you get the desired consistency.

-Pour the smoothie into the serving glass and serve chilled by sprinkling some cocoa powder on the top.

**Nutrition per serving**

Protein: 7g

Fat: 35g

Carbohydrate: 6g

# Banana-Berry Smoothie

Total time: 5 mins

Serves: 2

**Ingredients:**

- 3 tbsp. Golden Flaxseed Meal
- 10 drop Liquid Stevia
- 1 1/2 tsp. Banana Extract
- 1 tbsp. Chia Seeds
- 2 cups Vanilla Unsweetened Coconut Milk
- 1/4 tsp. Xanthan Gum
- 1/4 cup Blueberries
- 2 tbsp. MCT Oil

**Directions**

-Add all the ingredients in the blender and then wait for a few minutes so that the flax and chia seeds get time to soak some moisture.

-Blend them to form smooth paste and serve chilled.


**Nutrition per serving**

Protein: 4g

Fat:    25g

Carbohydrate: 3g

# Bomb of Fat Smoothie

Total time: 5 mins

Serves: 1

**Ingredients:**

- ½cup water
- 3 egg yolks
- ¼cup ice
- ½cup coconut milk
- 5 tbsp avocado
- Juice from lime or lemon

**Directions**

-Keep all the ingredients in the blender and then blend them to form a thick and smooth paste.

-Serve chilled.

**Nutrition per serving**

Protein: 11.7g

Fat: 51g

Carbohydrate: 12.4g

Fiber: 5.7g

# Ketogenic Strawberry Delight

Total time: 5 mins

Serves: 1

**Ingredients:**

- 3/4 cup Coconut Milk (from the carton)

- 1 tbsp. MCT Oil

- 1/4 cup Heavy Cream

- 7 Ice Cubes

- 1/4 tsp. Xanthan Gum

- 2 tbsp. Sugar-free Strawberry Torani

**Directions**

-Blend all the ingredients in a blender and make sure that you get the desired consistency.

-Serve chilled.


**Nutrition per serving**

Protein: 4.7g

Fat: 43g

Carbohydrate: 2g

# Choco-Blackberry Delight

Total time: 5 mins

Serves: 1

**Ingredients:**

- 7 Ice Cubes

- 12 drops Liquid Stevia

- 1/4 tsp. Xanthan Gum

- 1-2 tbsp. MCT Oil

- 1 cup Unsweetened Coconut Milk

- 2 tbsp. Cocoa Powder

- 1/4 cup Blackberries

**Directions**

-Mix all the ingredients in a blender.

-Blend them till all the ingredients are thoroughly incorporated.

-Serve chilled.

**Nutrition per serving**

Protein: 1g

Fat: 34g

Carbohydrate: 4g

# Cucumber Cooler

Total time: 5 mins

Serves: 1

**Ingredients:**

- 2 handfuls Spinach

- 12 drops Liquid Stevia

- 1/4 tsp. Xanthan Gum

- 1-2 tbsp. MCT Oil

- 2.5 oz. Cucumber, peeled and cubed

- 1 cup Coconut Milk (from carton)

- 7 ice Cubes

**Directions**

-Blend all the ingredients in a blender and make sure that you get the desired consistency.

-Serve chilled.

**Nutrition per serving**

Protein: 3g

Fat: 33 g

Carbohydrate: 4 g

# Smoothie-de-Tropics

Total time: 5 mins

Serves: 1

**Ingredients:**

- 7 Ice Cubes

- 20 drops Liquid Stevia

- 1 tbsp. MCT Oil

- 1/2 tsp. Mango Extract

- 1/4 tsp. Blueberry Extract

- 1/4 cup Sour Cream

- 2 tbsp. Golden Flaxseed Meal

- 3/4 cup Unsweetened Coconut Milk

- 1/4 tsp. Banana Extract

**Directions**

-Add all ingredients in a blender and wait for a few minutes. This will provide the flax meal with enough time to soak the moisture.

-Blend them to make a smooth paste and serve immediately.

**Nutrition per serving**

Protein: 5g

Fat:    31g

Carbohydrate: 3g

# Choco-Cream Shake (Ketogenic Version)

Total time: 5mins

Serves: 2

**Ingredients:**

- 16 ounces unsweetened almond milk
- 1/2 cup crushed ice (optional: add if you like a thick drink, but the flavor will be less intense.)
- 1 packet artificial sweetener
- 1 scoop Jay Robb Enterprises - Whey Chocolate Isolate powder
- 4 ounces heavy cream

**Directions**

-Blend all the ingredients in a blender and make sure that you get the desired consistency.

-Serve chilled.

**Nutrition per serving**

Protein: 15g

Fat: 25g

Carbohydrate: 4g

# Nutty Strawberry Smoothie

Total time: 2 mins

Serves: 2

**Ingredients:**

- 16 ounces unsweetened almond milk
- 1 scoop Jay Robb Enterprises - Whey Vanilla Isolate powder
- 1 packet artificial sweetener
- 1/4 cup frozen unsweetened strawberries
- 4 ounces heavy cream

**Directions**

-Keep all the ingredients in the blender and you can add some extra water to get the desired consistency after blending.

-Make sure to measure the strawberries as this recipe has slightly higher presence of carbohydrates in the ingredients.

-Serve immediately after blending.

**Nutrition per serving**

Protein: 15g

Fat:   25g

Carbohydrate: 7g

Fiber: 1g

# Cool Creamy Orange

Total time: 3 mins

Serves: 2

**Ingredients:**

- 16 ounces unsweetened almond milk
- 1/2 cup crushed ice (optional: add if you like a thick drink, but the flavor will be less intense.)
- 1 packet artificial sweetener
- 1 scoop Jay Robb Tropical Dreamsicle Whey powder
- 4 ounces heavy cream

**Directions**

-Blend all the ingredients in a blender and make sure that you get the desired consistency.

-Serve chilled.

**Nutrition per serving**

Protein: 15g

Fat: 25g

Carbohydrate: 4g

# Nutty Blueberry Delight Ketogenic Diet

Total time: 5 mins

Serves: 2

**Ingredients:**

- 16 ounces unsweetened almond milk
- 1 scoop Jay Robb Enterprises - Whey Vanilla Isolate powder
- 1 packet artificial sweetener
- 1/4 cup frozen unsweetened blueberries
- 4 ounces heavy cream

**Directions**

-Keep all the ingredients in the blender and you can add some extra water to get the desired consistency after blending.

-Make sure to measure the blueberries as this recipe has slightly higher presence of carbohydrates in the ingredients.

-Serve immediately after blending.

**Nutrition per serving**

Protein: 15g

Fat: 25g

Carbohydrate: 6g

Fiber: 1g

# Healthy Spinach Smoothie

Total time: 5 mins

Serves: 1

**Ingredients:**

* 1 cup unsweetened almond milk

* 50g spinach (about 2 handfuls)

* 10-15 drops of alcohol-free liquid stevia (optional)

* 1/2 cup full fat coconut milk

* 1 Tbsp MCT oil or coconut oil, melted

* 50g blackberries (about 10 berries)

* 1/2 scoop vanilla protein powder (I used Plant Fusion Vanilla)

* Small handful of ice

**Directions**

-Blend all the ingredients in a blender and make sure that you get the desired consistency.

-Serve chilled.

**Nutrition per serving**

Protein: 15g

Fat: 39g

Carbohydrate: 13g

# Keto Fruit-less Smoothie

Total time: 5 mins

Serves: 1

**Ingredients:**

- 1 cup unsweetened almond milk
- 1/2 scoop protein powder1 tsp cocoa powder
- 1 Tbsp hemp seeds
- 1 Tbsp MCT oil
- 1/2 avocado
- 1-2 cups spinach
- Ice cubes
- 1 tsp cacao nibs (optional)
- 10 drops liquid stevia
- 1/4 – 1/2 cup water for thinning out to desired consistency

**Directions**

-Add all the ingredients in a blender except the nibs of cacao and then blend them to form a smooth paste.

-Pour the liquid in the serving glass and sprinkle with the cacao nibs and serve immediately.

**Nutrition per serving**

Protein: 20g

Fat: 32g

Carbohydrate: 14g

# Keto Chocolaty Smoothie

Total time: 5 mins

Serves: 1

**Ingredients:**

- 20g NuZest Clean Lean Protein (Chocolate or Vanilla would work best)
- 1/4 cup full-fat organic coconut milk
- 8 drops liquid stevia
- 1 cup unsweetened almond milk
- 1/2 cup water
- 1/4 cup ice
- *1/2 Tbsp cacao powder if using vanilla flavour
- 50g avocado
- 1 Tbsp all natural peanut butter

**Directions**

-Blend all the ingredients in a blender and make sure that you get the desired consistency.

-Serve chilled.

**Nutrition per serving**

Protein: 23g

Fat: 31g

Carbohydrate: 6g

# Nutty-Fruity Vanilla Smoothie

Total time: 5 mins

Serves: 1

**Ingredients:**

- 1/2 Avocado

- 1/2 cup unsweetened vanilla almond milk

- dash of cinnamon

- no carb liquid sweetener to taste

- 1 tbsp almond butter

- 1/2 cup half and half

- optional: 1 scoop of vanilla Zero Carb Isopure

- splash of vanilla extract or sugar free vanilla syrup

- 3/4 cup of ice

- optional: Add fiber and omega-3's with 1 or 2 tablespoons of chia
  seeds

**Directions**

-First put all the liquid ingredients in the blender and then put the avocado,
almond butter and protein powder.

-Finally add the ice and then blend them together to form a smooth liquid.

-Serve immediately.

**Nutrition per serving**

Protein: 30.5g

Fat: 30.5g

Carbohydrate: 5.5g

# Ketogenic Coffee Shake

Total time: 5 mins

Serves: 1

**Ingredients:**

- 1 scoop vanilla Iso-Flex Isolate Protein Powder
- ¼cup of Greek yogurt
- Pinch of cinnamon
- 1 shot of espresso
- Pinch of stevia
- 5 cubes of ice

**Directions**

-Prepare the coffee and then put all the ingredients along with the protein powder in the blender.

-Blend them to form a smooth liquid and then serve immediately.


**Nutrition per serving**

Protein: 35g

Fat: 1g

Carbohydrate: 3g

# Raspberry Shake

Total time: 5 mins

Serves: 1

**Ingredients:**

- Raspberries (77g)

- Ginger (¼teaspoon)

- Strawberry protein powder (1 scoop)

- Almond milk (1 cup)

- Natural peanut butter (24g)

- ground coffee - (1 tablespoon) – optional

- Cinnamon (¼teaspoon)

**Directions**

-In the beginning you will add the almond milk with the raspberries in the blender and then add the whey protein powder along with natural peanut butter, ginger and cinnamon.

-Add the coffee if you want and then blend them together to form a smooth liquid.

-Serve immediately.

**Nutrition per serving**

Protein: 34.5g

Fat:    70.8g

Carbohydrate: 28g

Fiber: 12.1g

# Keto Smoothie-de-Avocado

Total time: 5 mins

Serves: 2

**Ingredients:**

- 1 ripe avocado

- 1/2 cup of ice cubes

- 1-2 tbps of your choice of sweetener

- 2 cups (480mL) of unsweetened almond milk

- few drops of vanilla extract

- 30ml of heavy cream (or whipping)

**Directions**

-Start by cutting the avocado into halves, remove the seeds and then scoop out the flesh in the blender.

-Now add the remaining ingredients and blend them together to foem a smooth liquid.

-Serve immediately.


**Nutrition per serving**

Protein: 3.5g

Fat:    23g

Carbohydrate: 9g

# Choco-Cream Splendor (Keto Version)

Total time: 5 mins

Serves: 1

**Ingredients:**

- Protein powder, low carb (under 3g carbs per serving), 25g (1 scoop)
- Sesame oil, 1 tbsp
- Liquid sweetener, 5 drops
- Cooking cream 35% fat, 100ml
- Psyllium husk, 1 tsp heaped (5g)
- Dark cocoa powder, unsweetened, 1 tsp (5g)

**Directions**

-Make a mixture of the protein powder along with the psyllium husk and cocoa and add 300ml water to shake the ingredients well. The psyllium husk will provide the necessary fibre.

-Now add the sesame oil and then the sweetener and shake again. The nutty flavour will be derived from the sesame oil and then add the cream, but do not shake.

-Serve by topping with some crushed ice.

**Nutrition per serving**

Protein:23 g

Fat: 52g

Carbohydrate: 6g

Fiber: 5g

# Ketogenic Shake-de-Protein

Total time: 5 mins

Serves: 1

**Ingredients:**

- 1 scoop Whey Protein Powder Vanilla (20 g)
- 6 drops of liquid stevia, vanilla flavored (or 1/2 packet of powdered stevia)
- 4 ice cubes
- 1 cup water (170 g)
- 2 Tbsp Heavy Whipping Cream (28 g)
- 1 oz Cream Cheese (28 g)

**Directions**

-Use an immersion blender to blend all the ingredients.

-Add the ice cubes and serve.

**Nutrition per serving**

Protein: 12.6g

Fat: 21g

Carbohydrate: 9.8g

Fiber: 4.5g

# Spinach' n' Cucumber Smoothie

Total time: 10-15    mins

Serves: 1

**Ingredients:**

- Spinach : Handful or 5 to 6 leaves, washed and chopped.

- Stevia ( any sweetener of your choice): 12 drops

- Mint leaves: 1 tsp chopped

- Cucumber : 1 medium size cucumber, peeled and chopped ( 1 cup)

- Coconut Milk : I used Dabur Homemade coconut milk ( 1 cup )

- Flax seeds (Alsi seeds) powder: 1tsp

- Coconut oil ( any MCT oil): 1tsp I used Patanjali Coconut oil

- Ice cubes

**Directions**

-Put the spinach in the blender and toss them.

-Now add the coconut milk and blend a little and then toss in the ice cubes.

-After this you will add the stevia and then the flax seed powder and the coconut oil and blend for few seconds.

-Stop the blender and let the ingredients to settle down and then blend again.

-After this the cucumber is to be added and blended. You can also choose to chop the cucumber and add it to the smoothie.

-Pour the smoothie in the serving glass and serve immediately by garnishing with mint leaves.

**Nutrition per serving**

Protein: 3.3g

Fat:    22.9g

Carbohydrate: 5.7g

Fiber: 2.7g

# Chocolaty Peanut Butter Shake

Total time: 2 mins

Serves: 1

**Ingredients:**

- 1 scoop choc. protein powder

- 1/2 Unsweetened Almond Milk

- 1 Tbsp Natural peanut butter

**Directions**

-Put all the ingredients in the blender and blend them to form a smooth liquid.

-If the paste is too thick, you can add some more almond milk to bring to the desired consistency.

-Serve chilled.


**Nutrition per serving**

Protein: 31.5g

Fat: 11.8g

Carbohydrate: 6.5g

Fiber: 1.5g

# Cheesecake and Strawberry Shake

Total time: 5 mins

Serves: 1

**Ingredients:**

- ½cup Strawberries, frozen, unsweetened
- 3 oz Philadelphia Cream Cheese
- 2 tbsp Philadelphia regular strawberry cream cheese,
- 4 tbsp Cool Whip whipped topping

**Directions**

-Blend all the ingredients in a blender and make sure that you get the desired consistency.

-Serve chilled.

**Nutrition per serving**

Protein: 7.3g

Fat: 36.1g

Carbohydrate: 18.8g

Fiber: 1.6g

# Ketogenic Protein Kahlua Shake

Total time: 5 mins

Serves: 1

**Ingredients:**

- 1 cup of water

- 3 tbsp of sugar free kahlua DaVinci syrup

- 2 cups of ice

- 1.5 tbsp of heavy cream

- 1 1/4 scoops of whey protein powder

**Directions**

-Blend all the ingredients in a blender and make sure that you get the desired consistency.

-Serve chilled.


**Nutrition per serving**

Protein: 33g

Fat: 10.8g

Carbohydrate: 3.1g

Fiber: 0g

# Protein Mocha Shake

Total time: 5 mins

Serves:1

**Ingredients:**

- 3/4 c water

- 2 Tbsp Kahlua DaVinci Syrup

- 1 Tbsp heavy cream

- 2 c ice

- 1 scoop chocolate protein powder

- 1 tsp instant decaf coffee

- 1/2 Tbsp unsweetened cocoa

**Directions**

-Blend all the ingredients in a blender and make sure that you get the desired consistency.

-Serve chilled.

**Nutrition per serving**

Protein: 27g

Fat: 7.9g

Carbohydrate: 5.3g

Fiber: 1.9g

# Roll of Cinnamon Smoothie

Total time: 3 mins

Serves: 1

**Ingredients:**

- 1 cup almond milk
- 4 teaspoons sweetener
- 1 teaspoon flaxmeal
- 2 tablespoons vanilla protein powder
- ½teaspoon cinnamon
- ¼teaspoon vanilla extract
- 1 cup ice

**Directions**

-Pour all the ingredients in the blender and then add the ice.

-Blend them together for 30 seconds and make sure that the liquid is smooth and thick.

-Serve immediately.

**Nutrition per serving**

Protein: 26.5g

Fat:    3.25g

Carbohydrate: 1.6g

Fiber: 1.1g

# Mint Delight Smoothie with Protein

Total time: 5 mins

Serves: 2

**Ingredients:**

- 1/2 avocado

- 1/2 cup unsweetened almond milk

- 1/4 teaspoon peppermint extract

- 1 cup fresh spinach

- 1 scoop whey protein powder

- 1 cup ice

- 10-12 drops of Peppermint Sweet Drops™

- Optional: cacao nibs

**Directions**

-Keep the avocado along with the protein powder, spinach and milk in the blender and blend them together to form a smooth liquid.

-Now add the Peppermint Sweet Drops extract and ice and blend till they form thick liquid.

-Taste and adjust the stevia if necessary and serve immediately.

Nutrition per serving

Protein: 20.7g

Fat: 13.3g

Carbohydrate: 9.4g

Fiber: 5.8 g

# Frappe-de-Choco-Mocha

Total time: 5 mins

Serves: 1

**Ingredients:**

- 2 cups unsweetened coconut milk

- 1 packet stevia (3.5oz)

- 1 packet instant coffee (about 2 tsp)

- 1 drop of coconut extract

- ½tsp unsweetened cocoa powder

**Directions**

-Take a large cup to mix all the ingredients and then stir them thoroughly to mix.

-Keep the mixture in a shallow freezer safe container and then scrape the mixture in every couple of hours with the fork.

-As the mixture becomes frozen you will then place on the counter and leave to soften.

-When it is soft, you will put it in the blender, blend for a few seconds and serve immediately.

**Nutrition per serving**

Protein: 0g

Fat: 10g

Carbohydrate: 2g

Fiber: 0g

# Green Salad Smoothie with Spice

Total time: 5 mins

Serves: 2

**Ingredients:**

- ½cup filtered water
- 1 handful fresh baby kale
- ½habanero pepper without seeds
- 1 lemon juice squeezed into blender
- 5 - 6 ice cubes
- 1 medium tomato, Roma or Heirloom
- ½Italian cucumber
- 1 cup of fresh white cabbage
- 1 handful fresh parsley

**Optional ingredients:**

- Dash of cayenne pepper
- 2 tablespoon of sunflower seeds

**Directions**

-Blend all the ingredients in a blender and make sure that you get the desired consistency.

-Serve chilled.

**Nutrition per serving**

Protein: 4.4g

Fat:   1.7g

Carbohydrate: 14.4g

Fiber: 4.2g

# Ketogenic Smoothie Splendor

Total time: 5 mins

Serves: 2

**Ingredients:**

- 2 eggs

- 1 pinch vanilla powder or vanilla extract

- ½cup (1 dl) blackberries,

- 3 tablespoons coconut oil

- ½cup (1 dl) full-fat yogurt, 10%

- ½cup (1 dl) water

**Directions**

-Use a stick blender to blend all the ingredients.

-Now add the flavour with some licorice powder or a piece of dark chocolate.

-Serve chilled or you can reserve it to serve later.

**Nutrition per serving**

Protein: 8g

Fat: 26.9g

Carbohydrate: 6.6g

Fiber: 1.9g

# Smoothie for the Breakfast

Total time: 5mins

Serves: 2

**Ingredients:**

- 100 g Ayam coconut milk
- 1/2 tsp vanilla extract
- liquid stevia to taste
- 50-100 g liquid of choice (water, coconut water, milk)
- 50 g frozen mixed berries
- 1/2 ripe avocado
- 10 g coconut oil
- 1 whole egg, raw (optional)
- 2 ice cubes

**Directions**

-Start by weighing the ingredients except the licorice and keep them in a mixing bowl.

-Use a hand blender to blend all the ingredients and then add the licorice of your choice.

-Serve chilled.

**Nutrition per serving**

Protein: 5g

Fat: 25g

Carbohydrate: 8g

# Paleo Smoothie

Total time: 5 mins

Serves: 2

**Ingredients:**

- 100 g raw, unsalted cashew nuts
- 4 ice cubes
- 1/2 ripe avocado
- 100 g frozen blueberries
- 300 g chilled water
- 1 tsp vanilla extract

**Directions**

-Put all the ingredients in a mixing bowl and blend with a hand blender.

-Serve chilled.

**Nutrition per serving**

Protein: 10.1g

Fat: 33.7g

Carbohydrate: 6g

Fiber: 5.8g

# Smoothie with Wild Berries

Total time: 5 mins

Serves: 2

**Ingredients:**

- 1 Egg

- 1 cup Frozen Berries

- 3 Drops Vanilla Essence

- 3 tablespoons Full Fat Yoghurt

- 100ml Cream

**Directions**

-Blend all the ingredients in a blender and make sure that you get the desired consistency.

-Serve chilled.

**Nutrition per serving**

Protein: 9.9g

Fat: 9.5g

Carbohydrate: 20g

Fiber: 2.5g

# Frosted Protein Shake Delight

Total time: 5 mins

Serves: 1

**Ingredients:**

- 2 cups ice

- 1 scoop chocolate protein powder

- 1 teaspoon instant espresso powder, dissolved in 2 tablespoon hot water

- 3/4 cup unsweetened almond milk

- 1/4 heavy cream

- 1/8 teaspoon liquid stevia

- 1 tablespoon cocoa powder

**Directions**

-Blend all the ingredients in a blender and make sure that you get the desired consistency.

-Serve chilled.

**Nutrition per serving**

Protein: 25g

Fat: 23g

Carbohydrate: 4g

Lightning Source UK Ltd.
Milton Keynes UK
UKOW01f2018140817

307301UK00008B/522/P